# If Only I Knew Then What I Know Now

*A Journey of Learning*

JOAN BERG

ISBN 978-1-64140-587-4 (paperback)
ISBN 978-1-64140-588-1 (digital)

Christian Faith Publishing, Inc.
832 Park Avenue
Meadville, PA 16335
www.christianfaithpublishing.com

Printed in the United States of America

# ACKNOWLEDGEMENT

I would like to thank my daughter,
Valerie Ramirez, for her assistance in writing this book.

# Raising Children

I cannot emphasize strongly enough the importance of this responsibility. The future of all the people which extend forward from this time will rely upon your decisions at this moment. In other words, how you raise your children is how they will raise their children and pass it on down through the generations. So now you can understand why your decisions at this time in your life are very important. With all these responsibilities that go with this challenge, let us focus first on the most important one. The most important gift that we can give our children is faith in God. As always, the Bible guides us to do what is right as can be read in the book of Matthew, "If anyone causes one of these little ones—those who believe in me—to stumble, it would be better for them to have a large millstone hung around their neck and to be drowned in the depths of the sea" (18:6, NIV). As you can see, the Bible tells us how important it is to raise our children loving and serving our God. How do we begin this path? First, let us teach our children how to pray each day and of course take them to church on Sunday to worship our Lord. Doing this for them throughout their youth will plant a seed. As they grow older they will carry on that tradition of attending church on Sunday, which gives them grace to believe and serve our God. You see, you can affect their lives so that they will lead good and Godly lives, which they will then pass on to their children and so on. This leads us into another important area in childrearing—discipline.

Discipline is a very important act as it teaches our children right from wrong which definitely gives them a conscience. For example, when we ask ourselves, "Shall I or shall I not do this?" and "Is it right or wrong?" When our children misbehave, disciplining them with love is very important even though they must know they're being disciplined. One of the no-no's in disciplining is anger. Never be angry with your children, for this teaches them how to be angry. Anger is not a good thing (if you read the Bible, you will know what it says about anger). If we could see ourselves in the mirror at the time that we are angry, think about what our children are looking at.

Now let's go into work of teaching our children. Another important part of raising children is teaching them well. One of the most vital things that we can teach them is compassion. Caring for the feelings of others is something that we need to learn at a very young age. This way, we stand back from teasing or bullying other children. We can show our children examples of how to be compassionate; for example, when a child is very upset and crying, you can teach your child how to comfort and, thus, help them feel better. In other words, befriend them when they are bullied by others as this can teach everyone who is watching to also have compassion. Another very important thought is something that we all must do; that is, to forgive. Our Lord tells us to forgive so we must teach our children to forgive. In other words, we must be an example as well a teacher. Following this path will point your children the way to heaven.

I would like to add a little pointer here that I learned through the years. When you ask your children to help you, add to your request that this is their responsibility and they will probably do their tasks more willingly. As the years go by and our children become teenagers, we certainly can be engulfed in a very difficult time. When our children go through these years, we find ourselves wondering how we can handle these problems for the children seem to be *on another planet.* So when we are going through this time, we must deal with our young adults with love and not with anger.

It has been long discussed that the brains of our children do not fully develop until about age twenty-five. Thus, we are essentially dealing with rather immature people who on the outside look like adults. I cannot stress enough that you should seek out guidance and help in doing the right thing for your children. Of course, we look to God for guidance at all times for He will help you and, as you well know, you cannot get better guidance than from our Lord. When we discipline our children through these young years, we do not want to damage them in any way. We say to our children as they graduate and go on with their lives, "Lead a godly life. This will take you to heaven when you leave this world."

# Teaching Children Respect

I imagine you are all familiar with the commandment, "Thou shall honor thy father and thy mother." Let us concentrate on the importance of this great commandment and let us understand the instructions our Lord has given us. Let us look at the book of Deuteronomy and read what our Lord is telling us to do: *"Honor your father and your mother, as the Lord, your God, has commanded you, that you may have a long life and that you may prosper in the land the Lord your God is giving you"* (5:16, NABRE). As we are growing up, especially when we become teenagers, we believe that we know everything and our parents know nothing. So we rebel against them when they try to guide us. In other words, we disrespect our parents in this way. Most of all, we must realize that our parents have lived much longer than we have lived and, furthermore, they have gained wisdom and knowledge throughout those years. They want so much to share this great knowledge and wisdom they have gained with their children. Unfortunately, more often than not, their guidance is rejected by the children who think they know everything. I believe very strongly that teaching children to be respectful to their parents needs to occur at a very young age. As a result, when they become teenagers they will not be totally shocked when *we come down on them* and address their poor choices and disrespectful behavior. Being taught respect during the early years will help prepare them to better accept discipline and guidance from their parents and elders rather than reject them so quickly. But always remember that thou shall honor thy father and thy mother.

# Think Before You Act

I would like to explore the consequences of making wrong choices in our lives. I think you have heard many ask the question, "Why me?" Let us go back to the day that we met the one we fell in love with and chose to marry. There were many warning signs that showed emotional problems in the one we married, but we chose to ignore such signs. As time goes on, we do have a wonderful wedding day celebrating with family and friends and a party that starts everything in a happy way.

After the party is over, we go on with our lives together. At first, things are relatively happy and we seem to have a good marriage. However, after a period of time, little by little, the emotional problems that we chose to ignore previously are beginning to resurface. But again, we chose to ignore. Then, as time goes on, there are children who enter into our lives and everything seems to be relatively okay.

However as time passes, the emotional negativity of our spouse becomes more significant and, consequently, more apparent.

That person becomes abusive, both mentally and physically. Not only does this abuse go to our spouse but also extends to the children. As a result, the marriage becomes an unhappy situation. As the children become older and go into teenage years, because of their own unhappiness in their home, they may resort to drugs and alcohol. These traits can become addictive. We then have other problems extending from the addiction which can cause many more problems. As you can see, our choice to ignore the warning signs before marriage have extended problems well into the future.

As our children grow older, they too may make the wrong choices in their marriages as a result of the suffering and unhappiness they experienced during the critical emotional developmental years. In actuality, this negative cycle of poor choices can go on indefinitely and be passed from generation to generation. Now you know how very important it is to choose the right person when you walk down that aisle to say, "I do."

We can go on with the "Why me?" scenario and consider another example of how making the wrong choice leads to hurting not only ourselves but others as well.

For instance, the weather report warns of icy roads, but we choose to get in our car and go where we intended, regardless. On the way there, we have an accident because of the ice, causing damage to two different cars and possible injuries to ourselves and the other people involved in the accident.

We now have significant problems because of injuries sustained and then recovery which can take a long time. We also have insurance payments, car repairs, and possibly law suits in our future. As much as the injuries we may have sustained may become permanent, we must also realize that the decision we made to drive on that icy day caused problems that extend far into the future. There are many other stories that can demonstrate consequences that result from making wrong choices, but these give you an example of what can happen when we don't stop to consider consequences. So let it be said, in the future, think before you act!

# SECTION 4

# Dedicated to Teenagers

When you are a teenager, you have a different view of the world around you. I do remember being a teenager. Those were the days when you knew everything; that time of your life when you thought you knew more than your parents, your teachers, etc. We all go through the teenage years and when you reach a much older age, you look back and you say to yourself, regrettably, "If I only knew then what I know now." So, I would like to propose a challenge to the teenagers who are reading this to carefully consider listening to your elders, rather than going through the pain caused by mistakes you can make as a young adult.

Admittedly, I did not listen to my elders when they tried to give me advice, but hopefully you will listen to advice from those around you who care. I'm going to present to you some old-fashion ideas—the ones that were right and kept you out of trouble. Because of the media we have today, they seem to think having sex is nothing more than just having sex, no commitments and no love. Sex can result in becoming pregnant. Now you have to make a choice of having a baby in your younger years and putting away all the plans you may have had to go to college and have a good career. Don't get me wrong, babies are beautiful blessings in our life and when you have a baby you know what love can be and how great it can be. But we first must get married, have security, and then bring into the world those beautiful children who you will love.

Let us go back and review what could happen if you make the wrong choices as a teenager. For example, taking drugs or drinking alcohol can have serious consequences. You can become addicted to these and, furthermore, contribute to making serious mistakes such as becoming pregnant with someone you hardly know, much less love. Even worse, you can contract sexually transmitted diseases.

All of these can become a significant dilemma in your life. Let's say you have this baby in which the father does not want to be responsible, the responsibility is yours and yours alone. You therefore, may not even be able to graduate from high school much less go to college. When you bring a baby into this world, you will experience a love like you have never known before. However, having this child should be at the right time under the right circumstances, such as having the needed security that a child requires to grow emotionally. The love from a mom and dad could be so beneficial to this young person.

Let us go to another scenario—the one that would be the right decision to make, such as graduating from high school, going to college, and becoming educated so that you can get employment that will be sufficient. Thereafter, you can find the right person that you will love and get married to. Choosing the right mate, as I had specified previously, is of the utmost importance because it can lead down two very different roads—a lifetime of happiness or a lifetime of unhappiness. Again, it's your choice and you alone can make the choices in your life that will bring about happiness for you and your children. But remember... it's YOUR choice!

Again, I would like to stress that when we are young, it is very difficult to distinguish between right or wrong or knowing which way you should go. Therefore, I cannot emphasize enough that you listen to your elders for their wisdom can help you make the right choices.

# Addiction

Now we will explore one of the most important issue of our times—drug and alcohol addiction. When we focus on these problems, we basically think of the individual and how it is affecting their lives and how they can be cured of their addictions.

Some seek rehabilitation in order to be cured or obtain some form of control over their addiction. Some achieve recovery during this time, but many others do not. Sadly, countless people continue to die from overdoses even following structured rehabilitation programs.

Addiction is so much greater than an individual's problem as its lasting devastating effects are felt by family and friends in many, many ways. Let us address this problem even further by looking into the future.

When a person abuses drugs and alcohol, the functions of the brain are altered and, furthermore, can become significantly damaged. Notably, research tells us that a person's social and emotional growth is stunted during drug abuse. In other words, when an adolescent takes drugs from the ages of fourteen to twenty-four, their emotional maturity is still the equivalent of age fourteen even though their age has increased.

When there is damage to the brain, affecting a person's ability to learn and ultimately achieve a meaningful education, what will our future look like? What will it become?

As the brains of our youth are being destroyed by drugs, who is going to be our future doctors, lawyers, politicians, and other community leaders?

As time goes on and cases of drug addiction increase, we will eventually have a multitude of people unable to function in our society. Ironically, the outcome of nuclear war can be compared to chronic drug addiction in our society, in that the eventual result is complete devastation and annihilation of our civilization, the former just having a faster result than the latter.

It is of the utmost importance that we support any actions that can be taken to prevent future addictions so that our youth can grow up mentally well and able to achieve a good education and become positive contributors to our world.

When we seek God to rid ourselves of drug and alcohol abuse, we can become everything we were meant to be according to His plan. Basically, when we look to God for help, we get help.

Therefore, we can conclude that addiction to alcohol and drugs are our greatest enemy and could destroy us as time goes on. Let us learn who the enemy is and let us then learn how to face and ultimately defeat that enemy. Only through God can we achieve this defeat!

# Depression

This section's objective is to reach out to the people who are suffering from sadness and despair to the deepest depths. This of course we know as depression, and even more severe, clinical depression. If, during periods of depression, people have thoughts of ending their lives, we can now understand that we must take action immediately. Of course, the first and foremost thing that we must do is trust in God's mercy and compassion. Through prayer and attending church, we can receive grace from God our Father, our Savior Jesus, and the Holy Spirit, which is food for the soul that enables us to move forward in Christ. Of course it is very important that you seek professional help from a doctor, preferably a psychologist, who is a doctor of the mind, who could be of great help to you. In as much as it is very challenging to identify the underlying causes of depression, a doctor can certainly help lead you in the right direction to feeling less pain and sorrow.

The very thought of someone taking their own life is so sad for the people who are left behind and love that person the most. It is so important to stop and imagine how devastating it will be to the people who love you the most when they hear of you taking your own life. So just when you think you are ending your pain and suffering, you are actually passing it on to those who love you, which they may feel for the rest of their lives. If you would think about this tragic picture before taking your life, perhaps you would change your mind and go on living. What a wonderful decision that would be for you and all the ones who love you. When you decide not to take your own life, you can think about things you can do in your life that are commendable, such as volunteer work, going to college, or even becoming a doctor and saving lives! Also, becoming a teacher and being a good example to them will help guide them to live productive lives. A teacher can have a lifetime effect on a child.

Along with these few suggestions, there are a multitude of things that you can do with the life that God has given you. Also, when you have found a reason to go on living and realize the thoughts that you had previously, you may be able to volunteer your time to help others who were in the same place that you were. I cannot express enough that you must think, think, and think some more before the act of taking your life because of the pain that you will inflict upon the people who love you.

# Dedicated to All of Those Who Ask the Question, "Why Do People Suffer?"

When we look around us, we see poverty, diseases, emotional anguish, etc. We, as humans, do not fully understand why such suffering is happening. Then we look to our Lord for answers for we know he is merciful, just, and loving, and, from here, we can seek further to find an answer to the question, "Why do people suffer?"

Let us look at the book of Matthew where Jesus describes the final judgment of nations.

> When the Son of Man comes in his glory, and all the angels with him, he will sit upon his glorious throne, and

all the nations will be assembled before him. And he will separate them one from another, as a shepherd separates the sheep from the goats. He will place the sheep on his right and the goats on his left. Then the king will say to those on his right 'Come, you who are blessed by my Father. Inherit the kingdom prepared for you from the foundation of the world. For I was hungry and you gave me food, I was thirsty and you gave me drink, a stranger and you welcomed me, naked and you clothed me, ill and you cared for me, in prison and you visited me.' Then the righteous will answer him and say, 'Lord, when did we see you hungry and feed you, or thirsty and give you drink? When did we see you a stranger and welcome you, or naked and clothe you? When did we see you ill or in prison, and visit you?' And the king will say to them in reply, 'Amen, I say to you, whatever you did for one of these least brothers of mine, you did for me.' Then he will say to those on his left, 'Depart from me, you accursed, into the eternal fire prepared for the devil and his angels. For I was hungry and you gave me no food, I was thirsty and you gave me no drink, a stranger and you gave me no welcome, naked and you gave me no clothing, ill and in prison, and you did not care for me.' Then they will answer and say, 'Lord, when did we see you hungry or thirsty or a stranger or naked or ill or in prison, and not minister to your needs?' He will answer them, 'Amen, I say to you, what you did not do for one of these least ones, you did not do for me.' And these will go off to eternal punishment, but the righteous to eternal life (Matthew 25:31–46, NABRE).

Now that we know what our Lord wants us to do in order to obtain eternal life, we have to look at those who are suffering and do as Jesus has asked—feed the hungry, clothe the naked, etc.—as indicated in Matthew's description of The Last Judgement. Now, if we reflect on the suffering of people, they are there for us to attend to and this is what God will judge us on during the final judgment.

If there was no one suffering, we could not fulfill what Jesus is asking us to do. Moreover, when people need clothing and we give it to them, we are fulfilling our Lord's will. If there was no hunger, who would we feed? If there was no nakedness, who would we clothe? If there was no one lonely or imprisoned, who would we visit and comfort?

Lastly, let us again realize that without the ones to comfort, clothe, and feed, we would not be able to fulfill services for the Lord in which we will be judged.

# Forgiveness

We shall now focus on forgiveness. It is one of the most important things that we can do for our own peace of mind. Let us go to an example of what I am trying to say. Let's say you go to work every day and there is someone in your office whose behavior causes you much stress and unhappiness. If you think about this, you will realize that another person's behavior is ruling your feelings of unhappiness and stress. When we give this much power to another person over us, we are now victims of our environment. When you go home in the evening, you carry with you this stress and your body suffers from this unhappiness. Try to understand that you do not have to take someone else's behavior upon yourself and suffer from it. That person is going about their lives unaware of your feelings and do not seem to be affected at all by the way their behaviors are affecting you. Therefore, would you not like to rid yourself of this burden and have peace and tranquility in your life? There is an avenue which you can take to help yourself achieve this and that is forgiveness.

Let's go back to our workplace where we have experienced a coworker who has caused us stress and emotional upset. Now, there are two ways that we can handle this situation. We can take on this person's behavior and cause it to be our own, or the alternative would be for you to reflect on forgiveness and forgive the person who is causing you emotional stress.

The end result of this action would be peace, which you will achieve if you take such a step. Now let's add this all up and see which is the best route to take. I'm sure that forgiveness will be your choice. When we find ourselves being unable to forgive completely what someone has done to us means that we have not used the correct approach in forgiving. When you focus on yourself being able to forgive, you do not have enough strength to do so. Therefore, when you forgive, forgive for God because God is the one who said we must forgive. When we choose to forgive for our God, we will be able to achieve that full forgiveness and peace at last. We do not fully realize the power of forgiveness until we have forgiven, and then we will reap the rewards such as knowing the peace that comes with forgiveness. To better understand how our Lord feels about you forgiving others who have hurt you, let's take a look at the book of Matthew as it will help you to understand more thoroughly how important it is to forgive.

*"If you forgive others their transgressions, your heavenly Father will forgive you. But if you do not forgive others, neither will your Father forgive your transgressions"* (Matthew 6:14–15, NABRE).

# Controlling Others

I would like to dedicate this section to something known as *control issues*. You may or may not have experienced such, so I will explain what I mean using the following example. Suppose a dear friend or loved one comes to you with an idea or plan that they intend to carry out, but you know doing such would likely cause them harm in one way or another. So you express strongly to them that what they are planning to do is a big mistake. For some reason, an overwhelming feeling of responsibility comes upon you and you become convinced that you must change their mind or you will bear partial (if not full) responsibility for their mistake. You actually convince yourself that you have an obligation to set this person on the *right* path as the outcome of their choice has now, somehow, been laid upon your shoulders. It is like you have now assumed a role in this person's destiny. Oftentimes, this intense need to control another person's behavior stems from feelings of unresolved *guilt*. In other words, a strong feeling of responsibility towards satisfying the best interest of another person sometimes stems from feelings of failure.

Now, if you were to approach this situation from another angle, you can simply offer your friend words of advice. You can humbly recommend something based on wisdom or just plainly what you believe is *the right thing to do* in such a situation. By gently guiding your friend using words of wisdom without heavy, emotional feelings of personal liability for the outcome, the ultimate decision is left with your friend, the owner of the problem. If your advisement is rejected, you cannot hold yourself responsible for the negativity that may come their way as a result of their decision.

Now, there is one way that we can be an active part of someone's destiny, and that is through prayer. For example, praying to our Lord for them to make the right decision. Now let me be clear that advising people of their mistakes is a good thing when it is done with patience and loving guidance.

Let me present you with another situation. Suppose you are a mother of three children and you go overboard cleaning and killing germs because if your children get sick it will be your responsibility (yet another guilt trip). Don't get me wrong, it is good to be clean—reasonably clean—for a household that is kept neat and clean is a very good thing for children. When we become neurotic about what we do, how clean we are, etc., then it becomes somewhat of a problem for you to live with.

# Can We Control Our Own Destiny?

When we focus on the concept of controlling one's destiny, we realize that the amount of control we actually have is miniscule. Using the weather, for example, will the sun shine? Will it rain? Will it snow? So when it concerns the weather, we have no trouble accepting that such is out of our control.

Let's explore this concept further using a young college graduate, for example, who decides to advance his academic career by attending medical school. After many years of hard work and studying, he achieved his goal in becoming a doctor. Now, he may think that he controlled his destiny through hard work and study. However, if we think about his road to success more deeply, he was born with a brain through no fault of his own, a brain with the ability to comprehend the rigorous studies needed to become a doctor. Our heavenly Father gave him this brain. God gives us life. Everything we have is because He has graciously given it to us and that includes a brain brilliant enough to pass all the tests necessary to become a doctor.

Let us further our venture into our family life. We have children who grow older each year and eventually become teenagers. We, as parents, have always felt that we were in control. However, at this time, we find we actually have little to no control over our teenager's behaviors and choices.

When our children go through this rocky stage of their lives, with all the hormonal changes that comes with it, parents start to experience great feelings of helplessness as they try to deal with the problems that exist. Even with such feelings of helplessness, parents continue to try to control destiny through many means, but with this we sadly forget that it is actually our Father in heaven who is in control, complete control.

We must look to our heavenly Father to guide us through the dilemmas we face and in doing so, in all meekness, we are turning all of our burdens over to God. Consequently, He then takes the reigns. Only then do we realize how little we control our destiny without the help of our Lord above. Let us now explore what the Holy Bible says about this subject using the Book of James. James offers Godly advice when we are faced with hardships, trials, etc., and proclaims that we should be rejoicing because of the spiritual gifts we will receive after. We are not to fall into hopelessness from such trials but rather we are to call out to our Lord, the one who gives so freely and lovingly, but with doing so we must relinquish all of our attempts to control along with every bad feeling that coincides. Basically, we cannot try to control while simultaneously giving it all to the Lord, as trying to do both is just senseless.

Consider it all joy, my brothers, when you encounter various trials, for you know that the testing of your faith produces perseverance. And let perseverance be perfect, so that you may be perfect and complete, lacking in nothing. But if any of you lacks wisdom, he should ask God who gives to all generously and ungrudgingly, and he will be given it. But he should ask in faith, not doubting, for the one who doubts is like a wave of the sea that is driven and tossed about by the wind. For that person must not suppose that he will receive anything from the Lord, since he is a man of two minds, unstable in all his ways (James 1:1–8, NABRE).

So you see, having full faith in what our Lord can do for us when we ask is a wonderful solution.

# A Letter to the Prisoners with Love

The following is a letter written for the prisoners to give them hope when they feel hopeless. Even though we have made the worst choices imaginable, know that our God is a forgiving God. You must never give up hope!

*A Letter to the Prisoners, With Love*

The purpose of this letter is to reach out to all the prisoners who are serving sentences in prisons around the country, some of which may be innocent of the charges that have been brought against them. Some of you may feel deep despair and a loss of any hope in your lives. That is why I would like to reach out to you and give you some inspiration as to why you are here on this planet. There is one thing we may wonder about. Is there a God who is up in heaven looking down upon us? I would like to share with you the proof that there is a God and that He does exist and most of all, He cares about you.

I have put together a demonstration of God's wonders—a picture of the universe. Sometimes, they say this all happened in one *Big Bang*, but if you carefully look at all the details of this great universe, you will see everything in a special place. For example, the earth sits at the correct distance from the sun so that life can exist. All the other planets and the stars remain in their place doing what they were meant to do, such as the Big Dipper. Notice that the stars that make up this particular constellation remain in place. We know this because they always form the image of a dipper. Thus, how could we question that this was not made by a greater being, a being far greater then we can imagine?

At this time, I would like to share with you a miracle that I was happy to witness. This miracle took place in 1959 in Washington, DC, where I was employed at the time. It was about three o' clock in the afternoon on Good Friday, the day and the hour that marks the anniversary that our Lord and Savior died on the cross for our sins over two thousand years ago. The sky began to turn darker and darker until it was black. It was a very strange event to have a black sky at 3:15 in the afternoon.

Everybody thought the world was coming to an end, but someone in the office told us that it would be back to normal at 3:30, which it was. Sometime later, I went into the Bible and read about this event. Saint Luke tells us that on the day that our Lord died on the cross, there was an eclipse of the sun. The black sky on Good Friday, 1959, was not a scheduled eclipse. That is, there was no scientific prediction of an eclipse of the sun to occur at that time. The following day, it was explained by the newspapers as an *unexplained phenomenon.*

I am sure that you have heard it said that God has no beginning and has no end. This statement is very difficult for us, as human beings, to comprehend. If you look up at the blue sky and try to see the end, you cannot imagine or comprehend an end. This gives us a visual understanding of God having no beginning and no end. With this, we can believe there is a God and then we can believe He loves us.

Now, we will go into passages in the Bible where Jesus explains just how much His father in heaven loves us—particularly the sinners as is seen clearly in the biblical story, *The Prodigal Son.* When Jesus spoke to the people, he spoke in parables. This way, the people could better understand the lesson that he was trying to teach.

Then he said,

A man had two sons, and the younger son said to his father, 'Father, give me the share of your estate that should come to me.' So the father divided the property between them. After a few days, the younger son collected all his belongings and set off to a distant country where he squandered his inheritance on a life of dissipation. When he had freely spent everything, a severe famine struck that country, and he found himself in dire need. So he hired himself out to one of the local citizens who sent him to his farm to tend the swine. And he longed to eat his fill of the pods on which the swine fed, but nobody gave him any. Coming to his senses he thought, 'How many of my father's hired workers have more than enough food to eat, but here am I, dying from hunger. I shall get up and go to my father and I shall say to him, 'Father, I have sinned against heaven and against you. I no longer deserve to be called your son; treat me as you would treat one of your hired workers.'" So he got up and went back to his father. While he was still a long way off, his father caught sight of him, and was filled with compassion. He ran to his son, embraced him and kissed him. His son said to him, 'Father, I have sinned against heaven and against you; I no longer deserve to be called your son.' But his father ordered his servants, 'Quickly bring the finest robe and put it on him; put a ring on his finger and sandals on his feet. Take the fattened calf and slaughter it. Then let us celebrate with a feast, because this son of mine was dead, and has come to life again; he was lost, and has been found.' Then the celebration began. Now the older son had been out in the field and, on his way back, as he neared the house, he heard the sound of music and dancing. He called one of the servants and asked what this might mean. The servant said to him, 'Your brother has returned and your father has slaughtered the fattened calf because he has him back safe and sound.' He became angry, and when he refused to enter the house, his father came out and pleaded with him. He said to his father in reply, 'Look, all these years I served you and not once did I disobey your orders; yet you never gave me even a young goat to feast on with my friends. But when your son returns who swallowed up your property with prostitutes, for him you slaughter the fattened calf.' He said to him, 'My son, you are here with me always; everything I have is yours. But now we must celebrate and rejoice, because your brother was dead and has come to life again; he was lost and has been found' (Luke 15:11–32, NABRE).

In this parable, we can see the great love of our Father in heaven has for us, as He forgives us readily for all our sins. Jesus spells this out for us in this parable so clearly. This parable demonstrates the rejoicing and celebration our Father in heaven has for us when we are genuinely sorry for our sins and ask to be forgiven. This is further verified when Jesus declared, *"…I tell you, in just the same way there will be more joy in heaven over one sinner who repents than over ninety-nine righteous people who have no need of repentance"* (Luke 15:7, NABRE).

God forgives us and rejoices over our repentance so we have no reason to doubt God's love and how much He is willing to forgive us. There are other passages in the Bible which will tell us the same thing as we just read as we surely know there is a gracious, loving, and merciful God in heaven who created the heavens, the earth, and all life.

Another great example of God's unconditional love and forgiveness is the story of Saul. Saul was a persecutor of Christians and yet God used him in a way where he actually became one of the greatest apostles found in the Bible.

Let us go back and try to review what has caused all of you to become incarcerated rather than being free. What kind of pain and suffering did you have to endure in your early life that may have contributed to the route you took, which ultimately led you to prison?

There are all kinds of different reasons for the actions that you had taken that put you behind bars, but let us think about what we can do to help make our future better.

Forgiveness is a giant word which means the difference between finding peace and happiness and not finding peace and happiness. As it is written in the Lord's Prayer, we ask God to forgive us for our trespasses as we forgive those who trespass against us. In other words, in order for us to be forgiven, we need to forgive. The Bible makes it quite clear as to how. One great example is to forgive for our sake as well as the sake of others. You say it's very hard to forgive. Yes it is. Without the grace of our Lord, we find it very difficult. When we follow God's law, we do it for God.

You may believe that your life is hopeless and that there is no future for you, but I want to remind you of when Jesus turned to Peter and stated, *"My kingdom does not belong to this world"* (John18:36, NABRE). Jesus was telling us how important our soul is and where we will go when we die, which can be with our Father in heaven forever. Forgiveness is one of the giant steps we can take to ensure our heavenly home is with our Father.

Over two thousand years ago, a man, an expert in knowing the law of the land, asked Jesus, *"Teacher, what must I do to inherit eternal life?" Jesus said to him, "What is written in the law? How do you read it?" He said in reply, "You shall love the Lord, your God, with all your heart, with all your being, with all your strength, and with all your mind, and your neighbor as yourself." He replied to him, "You have answered correctly; do this and you will live"* (Luke 10:25–28, NABRE).

Surely, we all want to go to heaven and be with God forever. Even though we may be sinners, the Bible tells us there is so much joy over the repentance of even one sinner.

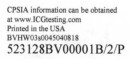

CPSIA information can be obtained
at www.ICGtesting.com
Printed in the USA
BVHW03s0045040818
523128BV00001B/2/P